KETOGENIC DIET

Weight Loss Mistakes to Avoid

Burn Fat Not Sugar

Achieve Rapid Fat Loss, Increase Mental Focus and Stay in
Ketosis

By
Wendy Williams

Table of Contents

Why You Need This Book

You feel a burst of energy inside and can go on for hours without thinking about food. You have stopped having hunger pangs, in fact you don't even remember the last time you actually felt them. Your mental focus has improved which helps you concentrate longer without feeling tired or irritable. Your body weight is in your control and you don't think about calories or weight loss while eating. You go to the gym or a hike not for losing weight but to feel good. You eat fresh and natural and know what's in your food. Whenever someone tells you about their weight loss problems you tell them how Keto has changed your life...

This is my story! And I believe it can be yours too.

But this was not always the case. I stumbled upon Keto by chance. And struggled to make this transformation a reality. A lot of research and trial and error has gone into reaching this sweet spot.

I know that plenty of people, including me, who have tried using Ketogenic Diet for weight loss but without proper guidance, have gone the wrong way. This prevents them from actually benefiting from ketogenic diet. The biggest problem is that there is too much half information and bad advice floating around. What is missing is a good framework to think about where we are going wrong or to assess if we are on the right track.

This book is written from my personal experience and anecdotal evidence from hundreds of fellow Keto Dieters who have helped me along on my journey. Through this book, my goal is to help you understand the core principles behind the Keto lifestyle and how to use them effectively for weight loss and improved health.

After reading this book you will be able to

- Assess your mistakes and correct them to get right back on track.
- Understand how Keto Diet actually helps you in weight loss.
- Appreciate that Keto Diet is a change in lifestyle and mindset.

When you are finished reading this book you will know more about human metabolism than your nutritionist or majority of the self proclaimed health experts.

Best of luck on your beautiful journey and I wish improved health and happiness to you!

I hope this book helps you in clearing all your Keto challenges. **Please leave a review once you finish reading**.

Now let's get started...

Why do we get Fat?

Volumes of books have been written on this subject. However, very few have actually been able to articulately explain the phenomena behind weight gain and obesity in a way that is simple and research backed at the same time. Lets try to explore the root cause of weight gain. The simplest explanation for this complex process is as follows....

When we eat starchy foods, like bread, pasta, potato or rice, our blood sugar (glucose) rises. Insulin, the hormone that regulates blood sugar, converts the excess sugar from the food into fat.

Since our body quickly digests carbs and sugar, the blood sugar levels decrease in a few hours causing us to feel hungry and crave for food again leading to binging and the vicious cycle continues. We end up burning sugars and accumulating fat resulting in weight gain.

This metabolic mechanism makes the carb centric diet detrimental for weight loss and increases the risk of diabetes. Let us explore further and understand how our body processes various macronutrients in a little more detail.

In the default metabolic state of high carb low fat diets, our body **burns sugar** and **stores fat**.

Energy in the body is extracted from Glucose, which is the fundamental source of energy for organisms and is the first nutrient to be used. Carbs are a direct source of glucose. Proteins can also be broken down into glucose by the body if required. However, the fat we consume is stored in fat cells as an energy reserve for later use. This fat storage is essentially our body's safety mechanism against starvation in case we run out of food.

When we consume food in a traditional diet

- Carbohydrates are broken down into Glucose. The energy derived from Glucose is used to fuel our bodily functions. A part of Glucose is also converted into fat by the insulin hormone and stored for later use.
- Dietary Fat is broken down into Fatty Acids. Human body is really good at storing fat. Fatty Acids from food are stored in fat cells which have unlimited capacity for storage.
- Protein is broken down into Amino Acids and used for vital functions like muscle building and transporting biological molecules. In case of shortage of energy, protein can also be converted into glucose and consumed.
- Sugar is broken down into Glucose and Fructose. Fructose is metabolised completely in the liver and is directly converted into fat.

As you can see, eating starchy and sugary foods encourage Fat storage. But Ketogenic Diet is the exact opposite. Carb and Sugar consumption is completely eliminated in the diet, so that our body starts burning the stored fat for energy. This helps in weight reduction and better health.

Ketogenic Diet:

A CHANGE IN PARADIGM

Ketogenic Diet is not a Diet in the usual sense of the word. It is a fundamental change in the way we think and make decisions about our food choices. Let me elaborate!

Do you remember Nicolaus Copernicus the great Renaissance Mathematician and Astronomer? In a time when it was widely believed that Earth is the center of the universe, this Polymath proposed a Heliocentric Model stating that sun is the center of the solar system. This led to a lot of controversy for a long time.

Ketogenic Diet is the Heliocentric Model of nutritional science. The conventional high carb low fat diet centers around carbohydrates and the use of glucose as the primary source of energy. Ketogenic Diet is a Low Carb High Fat diet that relies on Ketones derived from fat as the primary source for energy.

It is this contrarian view that challenges the premise of conventional dietary guidelines.

Ketogenic Diet in a Nutshell

In the fat burning Ketogenic Diet, carb consumption is restricted so the body is starved of sugar. Instead, greater quantity of Fat is consumed. Once the body detects this shortage of carbs, it starts burning the stored fat in the form of Ketones.

This triggers the state of Ketosis in which our body has a high fat-burning rate. Once this state is reached, Ketones are the primary source of energy for the body. So instead of burning sugar, our body burns stored fat for energy.

Proteins also play an important role in the Keto Diet. Some cells/organs in the body are unable to burn Ketones and need Glucose for energy resource. The amino acid in proteins are converted into glucose and fed to these cells.

The Inverted Food Pyramid

Easiest way to think about Ketogenic Diet is to imagine the FDA food pyramid and invert it. So now fats are the primary source of energy followed by proteins and carbs/sugar are completely eliminated.

Ketogenic Diet:

MORE THAN JUST WEIGHT LOSS

Ketogenic Diet is often thought of as a weight loss tool, which is only half the story. Weight Loss is of course one of the great benefits of a Keto Diet, and followers can lose up to three times as much weight as individuals on other diets according to studies [1]

However, it doesn't just stop there! Aside from weight loss, there are a whole host of other benefits for those who want to take control of their health using Ketogenic Diet! So let's have a look at how Keto Diet can improve a range of medical conditions and health issues.

Sharper Mental Focus

Individuals who follow Keto Diet will tell you that one of the great benefits is a feeling of razor sharp focus after perhaps years of mental 'fog' that a high carb diet can cause. This is because of the supply of essential fatty acids to the brain that are boosted as a result of Keto Diet. Followers also say that they experience increased energy levels on Keto Diet and are more motivated and focused to follow an exercise regime as part of the diet. A big plus all around!

Reduced Risk of Diabetes and Cancer

Metabolic syndrome is a cluster of conditions, mentioned below, that occur together. It is known to increase the risk of diabetes, stroke and cancer.

- Increased Fat in the Abdominal Cavity,
- High Blood Pressure,

- High Blood Sugar, and
- Lower levels of LDL (bad cholesterol)

Ketogenic Diet not only burns the fat stored in our body but also helps to regulate blood sugar by bringing down the insulin levels. This reduces risk of diabetes.

Sugar also feeds cancer cells. By reducing the blood sugar levels, the growth of cancer cells is restricted thus reducing the risk of cancer. [2]

Healthier Heart

We all know that a healthy heart is essential for a healthy body. Low carb eating has long been touted as a great way to lower blood pressure and also improve overall cholesterol levels in followers. As Franziska Spritzler, a registered low carb dietitian says:

"People who restrict carbohydrates and increase intake of healthy fats like olive oil, coconut oil, butter, lard, tallow, avocado, olives, and nuts almost universally experience a drop in triglycerides and an increase in healthy HDL cholesterol." [3]

The reason for this is that the more fats we eat, the more HDL cholesterol (also known as 'good cholesterol') our bodies produce. Not only is HDL cholesterol good cholesterol, it is also linked to decreased levels of heart disease.

You Feel Sated!

Yes! This is one of the great benefits of Keto Diet, as fatty foods are the most sating of all the macronutrients. So the hunger pangs that we experience from a carb loaded diet is completely eliminated.

The followers of Keto Diet stay fuller for longer and thus tend to eat less than individuals on other diets. This decreased appetite, or feeling fuller for longer, in turn leads to increased weight loss.

This makes Keto Diet a sustainable way of weight reduction. As opposed to other conventional diets that often leave followers feeling hungry and thus unable to stick to them for a long time.[4]

Fat Loss from the Abdominal Cavity

Remember- not all fat is the same. The place where fat is stored on your body can have a dramatic effect on your overall health as well as the kinds of diseases that you may be prone to.

Fat can be either subcutaneous which means that it is lodged under the skin, or visceral, which means it is stored inside the abdominal cavity. The latter is one of the worst places our body can store fat as it ends up around our organs. This leads to a whole host of issues like inflammation, resistance to insulin, and dysfunction of the metabolism. The good news with Keto Diet is that most of the fat loss will be around the abdominal cavity, thus decreasing all of these risks. [5]

Natural Treatment for Alzheimer's Disease

One of the main causes of disorders such as Alzheimer's disease is the brain's increased resistance to insulin. This is because neurons in the brain use glucose, as their main source of energy, and diets that are high in carbohydrates are known to produce elevated levels of glucose and insulin in the body.

If the levels become too high however, the brain builds up a tolerance and resistance to insulin, and begins to shut down as it is starved of essential energy for the neurons.

Where Ketogenic Diet can help patients is in lowering carbohydrate intake, which means that the body produces ketones instead of glucose. Instead of being fed by glucose, the brain is fed by ketones and when this happens it reduces brain related issues such as Seizures, Alzheimer's Disease, and Parkinson's Disease.

Another way in which Keto Diet can be used as a treatment for Alzheimer's disease, is through the increased intake of coconut oil which is packed with fatty acids that are immediately turned into fuel by the body and provide much needed energy for the brain. [6]

Reduced Risk of Fatty Liver Disease

The primary cause of fatty liver disease is Fructose and Alcohol. When you consume these two toxins, they are metabolised by the liver and stored as fat inside the liver. Over a period of time, the fat accumulation leads to fatty liver disease.

Studies undertaken at Duke University have shown that Ketogenic Diet can work wonders when it comes to the fatty liver disease. The natural food groups included in the diet help you stay away from all the classic problem foods, Alcohol and Fructose, associated with a Fatty Liver Disease. [7]

Keto Diet Mistakes

Now let's look at the top mistakes Keto Dieters make and strategies to overcome them. It is helpful to keep them in mind even after you are successfully leading a Keto Lifestyle.

Mistake 1:

NOT KNOWING YOUR MACRO PROPORTIONS

Ketosis is a reversible phenomenon. So long as you are using fat as your primary food and burning ketones for energy you will be able to control your weight and blood sugar levels. As soon you switch back to carbs, eat too much of proteins or reduce the proportion of fat in your diet, the body goes back to burning sugar for energy.

That's why maintaining an optimum proportion of Fats, Proteins and Carbs in your diet is so important for a Ketogenic Diet. Majority of the people falter in keeping this balance of proportion in a sustainable way over a long period of time.

So what is the Optimum Proportion?

Again, the answer to this question is more nuanced than you would like to hear. In short the answer is, **Know Your Own Body**. Please find the recommended ranges below, but you will have to work with your body to determine the optimum amounts suitable to keep you in Ketosis.

In terms of percentage ratio the following proportions are recommended.

- Fat 60-75%
- Protein 15-30%
- Carbs 5-10%

Broadly the proportion depends on the following factors.

- Your Body Mass Index
- Your Age
- Your Percentage Body Fat
- Your Activity Level

If you are **just starting** on your Keto Diet, it's best to restrict your carb intake to **20-30 grams per day** (remember 1 big orange = 1 pint of beer = 20 grams carb). For majority of the people, carb intake range can be increased to **20-50 grams per day** once you have achieved the desired weight loss and are in the **weight maintenance phase**.

There are number of Keto Calculator Apps you can find that will help you in calculating your exact macro proportions. [8]

Mistake 2:

SCALE WATCHING

You need to accept the fact that being on a Keto Diet is a lifestyle change and not a crash diet. You will get there, keep calm and carry on!

It's natural for you to want to weigh yourself regularly to check progress when on a diet, but this is actually not a very accurate way to measure results. You need to realise that weight is just a number and is neither a very meaningful or accurate measure of how you are progressing nor an indicator of fat loss or physical fitness. Just remember that apart from your water weight that can fluctuate several pounds in a short span, the scale is a snapshot of what happened two weeks back.

What is the difference between your friend who weighs 300 lb. and an athlete who weighs the same? They do weigh the same but is their body composition the same?

It is important to understand that losing fat and weight are two different things. As we lose body fat and gain muscle mass especially for someone who has recently begun exercising, the scale would continue to show the same weight.

Indicators that you are on track to losing weight even if the scale doesn't budge

- Your tape measurements show a shrinking waistline
- Your clothes are getting looser, you look slimmer, and people around you notice the difference.
- You have lots of energy and want to exercise after living a sedentary lifestyle for years.

- Your health markers are improving.
- Your Body Mass Index (BMI) dips.
- Your mental focus improves, you don't experience afternoon slumps anymore.

Measure your Ketones

Measuring ketones is a good way to know that you body is in Ketosis and is burning the stored fat. There are a number of ways to measure ketones produced in your liver as your body goes through ketosis. These include urine test kits, blood test kits, breathalysers, and good old-fashioned observation techniques. Depending on your budget and interest, measuring ketones can be a good way to monitor results during ketogenic diet.

Mistake 3:

SUGAR ADDICTION

Sugar is the biggest hindrance to leading a healthy lifestyle. Removing sugar completely from your diet is absolutely necessary for a successful transition to Ketogenic Diet lifestyle. In fact, a gradual removal of this single substance from your diet alone will make you healthier than majority of the people. If you want to take one lesson from this book it is to completely remove sugar from your life.

The average per capita sugar consumption in America has risen to 153 grams per day from 9 grams per day back in 1822. Our bodies have got so used to sugar that in reality it is difficult to get through a day without consuming sugar in some form. Being so readily available and ingrained in our lifestyle makes it all the more difficult to give up sweet foods. Check out the Resources section of the book for **56 different names of sugar** used by the processed food industry to hide the amounts of added sugar in your food.

You often hear justifications in favour of sugar consumption, like ......

"It's okay to consume everything in moderation"

"It is needed by your body"

"A little bit will not harm"

Let us try and understand if there is any truth in the above.

So what is Sugar?

Sugar is simply Glucose + Fructose (The Sweet Part). It has

- No healthy fats

- No protein
- No vitamins
- No enzymes

How Sugar makes us Eat More!

Sugar triggers a chain reaction where high levels of sugar in the bloodstream results in increased insulin levels. This insulin in turn makes it difficult for the brain to receive the satiety signal. As a result the brain is fooled to believe that the body is still hungry leading to excessive food consumption and weight gain.

How to Overcome Sugar Cravings

- **Reduce your Carb Intake:** A high carb diet causes blood sugar to rise, which in turn signals the body to release insulin. You need to increase your consumption of protein and good fat to overcome this. Proteins are made up of amino acids, which are important for balancing hormones and sugar cravings. Healthy fats are a source of energy for our body and help reduce hunger pangs and provide satiety.

- **Plan Your Meals in Advance:** Hunger is not the best time to make rational decisions on what is best to eat. Planning ahead to include nutrient rich food in your diet will help curb hunger swings and sugar cravings.

- **L-Glutamine:** Dr. Julia Ross in her book *"The Mood Curse"* suggests that intense sugar cravings are due to stress, poor diet and deficiency of amino acids (to the extent that diet alone may not be able to correct it). She suggests a short-term supplementation of amino acid L- Glutamine.

- **Check your Pantry:** Keep sugary foods out of sight as much as possible.

- **Watch Out for the Hidden Sugar:** Low fat, sugar free and diet foods contains added sugar or synthetic sweeteners in order to enhance the taste of the food and palatability. Get into the habit of going through the labelling for savoury foods, juices, sauces, salad dressings and condiments. You will be surprised how many of them contain sugar.

- **Avoid Artificial Sweeteners:** Replacing sugar with a sugar substitute in the belief that it will reduce calorie intake and help in weight loss is a myth. Recent studies have shown that on the contrary artificial sweeteners maintain the cravings for sweet food and increase appetite.

Our body increases insulin secretion in anticipation that sugar will appear in the blood stream. When the body doesn't receive the sugar, insulin uses the existing sugar in the bloodstream for energy. As a result, blood sugar levels drop and hunger increases leading to uncontrolled binging.

Mistake 4:

ELECTROLYTE IMBALANCE

Electrolytes are salts that flow in your blood stream and carry an electric charge. They are essential for the cells in our body to function properly, whether it is to regulate blood pressure, help with muscle contraction or nervous system functions.

It is a well-known fact that on a Keto Diet the initial transition phase results in significant water loss. With the water are lost essential minerals like sodium and potassium, which triggers an electrolyte imbalance.

You will need THREE TIMES more electrolytes when on a Keto Diet as compared to a normal diet.

Signs that you have an Electrolyte Imbalance

- You are restless, have muscle aches, spasms and joint pains
- You have heart palpitations and find it difficult to sleep.
- You experience dizziness and fatigue

Important Electrolytes Include

- **Sodium**: Responsible for maintaining fluid balance in our bodies, helps in muscle contraction and nerve signalling.

  Sources: Table Salt and Himalayan Pink Salt.

- **Magnesium**: One of the most under-appreciated minerals, Magnesium helps in maintaining a stable heart rate, bone building, creation of DNA and RNA and normal nerve and muscle functions.

Sources: Almond, Salmon, Spices and Leafy Veges.

- **Potassium**: It aids muscle contraction, regulates heart contractions and keeps blood pressure stable. An imbalance of sodium and potassium is caused when we consume sodium loaded processed foods and skip vegetables rich in potassium. This could lead to hypertension, heart attack and stroke.

  Sources: Avocado, Nuts and Dark Leafy Veges.

- **Calcium**: In addition to helping with formation and maintenance of bones and teeth, calcium helps with cell division, cell clotting and transmission of nerve impulses.

  Sources: Almonds, Cheese and Broccoli.

Healthy individuals who are not working out extensively get their daily intake of electrolytes from the food they eat. However if you are sick, out on a very hot day or on a low carb diet, your electrolyte requirement spikes up.

Homemade Keto Friendly Electrolyte Drink

Time to Preparation: 5 Minutes

Source: http://ketodietapp.com/Blog/post/2015/10/19/beat-keto-flu-with-homemade-electrolyte-drink

Ingredients

- 5 cups water
- 4 fl oz lemon juice
- ½ tsp potassium chloride *or* lite salt
- ¼ tsp pink Himalayan *(or to taste)*
- 2 tbsp Natural Calm magnesium supplement

Instructions

- Juice the lemons
- Place ingredients in a jug and stir until combined.
- Add some ice cubes and serve.

Mistake 5:

FAT PHOBIA

For years we have been told that *eating fat will make you fat*. Some of the most popular diets in the world are based around this premise. It is this social conditioning that leads us to subconsciously make choices that are low in fat. As a result sugar and grains have been the primary source of the calories for most of us. Once you remove these two from your diet you will need to replace them with another energy source. If you don't you will feel hungry, tired and low all the time and will eventually switch back to carbs.

It is important to understand that there are two sources of energy – glucose and ketones. When on a low carb diet, sufficient intake of fat (60-75 % of total intake) leads us into ketosis and our body uses ketones for energy. However if our body does not get into ketosis, it will look out for glucose for energy. It will either get it from carbohydrates or from protein (through Gluconeogenesis).

Keto Diet advocates a mix of **saturated fats, omega 3s and monounsaturated fats**.

Different types of Fat Present in our Food

- **Saturated Fat (SFA)**: They are stable fats, with long shelf life and suitable for high flame cooking. They help keeping in check your bone density, immune system and testosterone levels. Contrary to popular belief their consumption does not adversely affect the heart.

  Sources of SFA: Meat, Egg, Butter, Ghee, Lard, Coconut Oil are good sources of Saturated Fat.

- **Monounsaturated Fat (MUFA):** They are liquid at room temperature and best for cold use for salads or after cooking. Good for the heart, they are now a popular choice of fat.

  Sources of MUFA: Avocado, Olives and Nuts (especially macadamia).

- **Polyunsaturated Fat (PUFA):** This type of fats can be primarily divided into the naturally occurring Omega 3s and the industrially processed Omega 6 fats. PUFAs are unstable and fragile and not suitable for cooking. When heated, they react with oxygen to form harmful compounds called free radicals, which in turn raise our risk of heart diseases and cancer. Omega 3 consumption is good for our body but most of the PUFA cooking oil is high in omega 6, which is harmful.

  The ideal ratio of Omega 6 to Omega 3 fats is 1:1. However in reality the ratio is way higher than this, ranging from 10:1 to 20: 1 on a average, so not only do we have a problem of excess Polyunsaturated fat, we also have much higher proportion of omega 6 fats and deficiency of omega 3s.

  Sources of healthy Omega 3s: Wild Salmon, Walnut, Fermented Cod Liver Oil, Macadamia Nuts and Grass Fed Meat.

- **Trans Fat:** This is considered as the **worst form of fat** and should be avoided. Trans fat is unsaturated fats primarily found in processed foods where through industrial process hydrogen is added to liquid vegetable oil to cause the fat to become solid at room temperature. This partially hydrogenated oil helps increase the shelf life of processed food. It is linked to heart diseases and has an adverse effect on cholesterol levels.

  Stay clear of products whose product label mentions words like "trans fat", "hydrogenated". It is worth noting that in United States if a product has less than 0.5 grams of trans fat per serving then the label can say 0 grams of trans fat. These hidden trans fat quickly add up if you consume multiple servings.

High Fat Foods to Include in Your Diet

- **Avocados:** Avocado unlike most fruits is loaded with monounsaturated fat oleic acid. This is the main fatty acid in olive oil and linked with various health benefits. It is a great source of potassium and fibre and helps lower triglyceride.
- **Cheese:** It is made from milk of grass fed animals is a good source of nutrients as it is high in saturated fats and omega 3-s, protein and amino acids
- **Whole Eggs:** Eggs are one of the most nutrient dense foods and are loaded with vitamins and minerals.
- **Fatty cuts of Meats and Fish:** Include fatty cuts of grass fed animals. Avoid chicken breasts or lean meat where the fat has been removed. Include fish like Salmon, Sardine, Mackerel and Trout in the meal plans. If you cannot eat fish then it is worth considering a supplement like Cod fish liver oil, which contains Omega 3-s and Vitamin D.
- **Nuts:** Nuts are loaded with Protein, Vitamin E and Magnesium in addition to healthy fats and are a great option to add to a meal when consumed in moderation. Almonds, Walnuts and Macadamia nuts are some of the healthy choices.
- **Chia seeds:** They are high in Omega 3 fatty acids and Fibre. They can be a useful addition to your diet
- **Extra Virgin Olive Oil:** Rich in vitamin E & K and loaded with antioxidants, extra virgin Olive oil is an excellent choice. The antioxidants in the oil helps in improving cardiovascular health, lower blood pressure, fight inflammation and protect LDL particles from oxidation in the blood.
- **Coconut Oil:** It contains 90% saturated fatty acids making it the richest source of saturated fat.
- **Butter and Ghee (clarified butter):** Butter has been demonised for long but Grass Fed butter is good for you. In addition to Vitamin A, E and K2 it contains Conjugated Linoleic Acid (CLA) and Butyrate. CLA helps in lowering fat percentage and Butyrate improves the gut and fights inflammation.

- **Lard, Tallow and Bacon** Fat from naturally raised animals are a great option for cooking and are high in healthy saturated and monounsaturated fats

What to Avoid

- Vegetable and Seed oils rich in omega 6s
- Artificial trans fats
- Hydrogenated fats like margarine

Mistake 6:

CARB LOADED

So much has already been discussed about carbs. But I would like to reiterate that you should become aware about your carb tolerance. An athlete will probably have a greater carb tolerance than someone with a sedentary lifestyle. On the safer side, your carbs intake should not go beyond 20 grams max when you start your Keto Diet.

Getting rid of carbs may work in the short term, but there always comes a time when all of us start to crave for the starchy stuff. The temptation of having just that one small slice of bread can be overwhelming.

Let me warn you again though, **Ketosis is a reversible state** and can be broken very easily by just having that one small piece. Not only that, once you start eating that one piece, insulin level in your blood starts to rise which will play all kinds of havoc with you. Let us understand how a high carb diet affects us physiologically.

Why "Eat Less and Exercise More" in Not a Solution

The conventional weight loss wisdom from the diet industry is 'Eat less and Exercise more'. This advice, derived from the calorie in calorie out (CICO) theory, falls flat in the world of complex human physiology. CICO completely ignores the inner workings of a human body and has led to lots of people abandoning their weight loss quest.

People who propagate CICO believe that **Calorie IN = Calorie OUT + Stored Fat**. So the amount of fat stored in the body depends upon the amount of calories we consume minus the calories expended in bodily functions and exercise. Nothing can be far from the truth!

Human body has no way of measuring calories but has its own way of regulating fat. Insulin is the hormone that controls how much energy we expend and how much is stored as fat.

When we eat, the insulin goes up and body starts storing fat. And eating equal calories of carb will raise insulin level more that eating equal calories of fat. That's why in human physiology; a **calorie is not a calorie**. As we stop eating, the insulin level drops and body stops storing fat. As the fasting continues body starts burning the stored fat.

That's why conventional (High Carb Low Fat) diets fail. Because of high insulin levels in carb-based diets, fat is being continuously stored. So even if you are eating lesser calories overall, insulin levels will remain high because of carb consumption and fat storage will continue. Ironically, weight gain continues and with increased appetite.

In a Low Carb High Fat (LCHF) diet however, the insulin levels are lower. So when you consume equal calories of fat based food, a part of your energy needs will be met with the stored body fat. So using a LCHF diet for fat loss is more effective as your appetite is decreasing with a steady decline in body fat.

Mistake 7:

EXCESSIVE DRINKING

Keto Diet does not mean the end of your social life. Sure hit the bars, but you have to do so responsibly. Please remember if it tastes sweet, it's probably sugary and should be avoided.

You will have to keep a check on what you drink and how much you drink. Beer and wine should be especially avoided as they contain a lot of carbs and sugar.

When you consume a drink your body will metabolize it on priority before other sources of energy, as it cannot store alcohol. This means that although alcohol consumption will not completely throw you out of ketosis it will for sure prolong the timeline for your goals. This is because when the body is burning alcohol for energy it is unable to metabolize the stored fat.

Remember to drink plenty of water in between your drinks. Keto lowers your alcohol tolerance level so keep sufficient gap between drinks.

Unsure of what to drink and what to avoid?

Lets look at the carb contents of various alcohols to get you started.

Spirits

- Unsweetened Spirits are Zero Carb: Whiskey, Scotch, Vodka, Gin, Rum, Brandy, Tequila, Cognac. 96 calories PER SHOT.
- Liqueurs have sugar: Jagermeister, Vermouth , Amaretto, Curacao, Grand Marnier, Cordials, Limoncello. Although

these usually are not had by themselves but are part of several cocktails.

- Mixers: Try and mix the spirits with diet soda or simply water to keep out the carbs from your drink. Avoid tonic as it has both carbs and sugar!
- Martini: Go for extra dry when it comes to martini as dry vermouth has carbs. Although a few drops won't harm.

Wine

Wines need to be considered on a case-by-case basis. Dessert wines, ports, and Sherries are sweetened and should be avoided.

Here is the nutritional value for a serving of 5 ounce

Red Wine

- Cabernet: 120 cal, 3.8g carbs
- Pinot Noir: 121 cal, 3.4g carbs
- Merlot : 120 cal, 3.7g carbs

White Wine

- Champagne/Sparkling whites: 96 cal, 1.5g carbs
- Chardonnay : 118 cal, 3.7g carbs
- Pinot Gris/Grigio: 122 cal, 3.2g carbs
- Riesling : 118 cal, 5.5g carbs

Beer

Sorry but majority of the drinks here are high calorie and high carb. Although light beers maybe fine to drink avoid drinks that are dark, amber, or red.

Here is the nutritional value for a serving of 12 ounce

- MGD 64 : 64 cal, 2.4g carbs
- Michelob Ultra : 95 cal, 2.6g carbs
- Bud Select 55 : 55 cal, 1.9g carbs
- Coors Light : 102 cal, 5g carbs
- Miller Lite : 96 cal, 3.2g carbs
- Natural Light :95 cal, 3.2g carbs

- Rolling Rock Green Light : 92 calories, 2.4g carbs
- Bud Light : 110 calories, 6.6g carbs
- Bud Select : 99 calories, 3.1g carbs
- Michelob Ultra Amber : 114 calories, 3.7g carbs
- Amstel Light : 95 calories, 5g carbs

Mistake 8:

SURRENDER TO TEMPTATIONS

One can have no smaller or greater mastery than mastery of oneself.

—Leonardo Da Vinci

Learning to say no, to yourself and to others, is one of the most useful skills to develop when it comes to living a healthy life. Even small changes can make a huge impact. Maintaining a Ketogenic Diet will be a test of your grit. There will be situations everyday when you will need to say no to something.

For example: your friend offers you a dessert and you are tempted to say yes, or your office party has only beer and pizza and everyone is asking you to have something.

To put it simply: you can either choose to play victim or overcome temptations.

Which one would you prefer?

Control Your Environment

Starting a new habit is not easy and breaking bad ones can be even more challenging.

How do you make it easier for yourself to break bad habits, say no and resist temptations?

One change you can make right now is to Control Your Environment. The environment that you live in makes it easier to adopt bad habits and difficult to keep good ones. This is the reason why it's so damn hard to break old habits and stick to new ones, even if you consciously want to make a change.

You are not alone; we all have driven the same road. Here's what you can do about it...

Out of Sight, Out of Mind

When I started on my Keto journey, I could not stick onto the diet for more than a few weeks. The intention and the motivation was all there. I would plan everything and make all the right choices but after a few days of doing things right, I would just fall off. It was really depressing.

This happened four times but then I noticed that many of the actions I took were simply a response to the way things were organized around me.

For example, I love cookies. Whenever I went to the pantry I used to pick a few. I did this not because I craved for a cookie but because I was simply responding to the environment around me.

After a few observations, I started to redesign my environment. The first thing I did was to bin all the carbonaceous foods and sugary drinks at home and replaced my kitchen with cheese, coconut oil, nuts and all kind of natural fatty foods. That way, when it was time to eat, I see them sitting right there in front of me.

The idea is to make habits you want to perform more visible and the habits that you don't want to perform less visible.

Mistake 9:

EXERCISE TO LOSE WEIGHT

The common belief is that we exercise to lose weight, stay fit and build muscle and strength. Let us try and understand if exercise really helps in weight loss.

Before I started my journey on low carbs I used to spend a couple of hours everyday exercising. I did rigorous cardio sessions with the aim of losing weight and staying fit. My aim was to lose 20 pounds and I believed that exercise would take me there.

To my disappointment even after a month of rigorous exercise, the scales just didn't move! Despite what seemed at that point the holy grail of weight loss I felt exhausted and hungry.

It was only later when I researched in depth that I realised; aiming for fat loss on a calorie-restricted diet along with rigorous exercise simply does not work.

Prolonged cardio makes you hungry and leads to overeating. It also makes you physically and mentally exhausted.

Why Cardio Does Not Help in Weight Loss?

- Cardio makes you hungry and unless you force yourself not to eat, you will binge. Most of the time you will crave for comfort food that will pack on extra pounds.
- When doing rigorous exercise, your stress levels rise and with that the stress hormone cortisol is released. This results in visceral fat accumulation on your abdominal area. Cortisol (the stress hormone) also suppresses the signals of the satiety

hormone leptin, which again will make you eat more and you wouldn't know when to stop.

- Regular intensive cardio can lead to chronic inflammation. Effective exercise does cause inflammation, which is actually necessary for muscle building and improving performance. As long as the body resolves the inflammation response quickly it does not harm. However when the stress associated with the inflammation is not removed (caused again and again every single day) chronic inflammation develops.

To conclude a change in mindset is needed here. There are no one size fit all answers to what would be the right exercises to do. Instead my advice is that you should not exercise to burn calories and lose weight. Instead do it for pleasure, to build muscles and feel good.

Mistake 10:

IMPORTANCE OF PROTEINS

Like many of us do you also have the notion that Ketogenic Diet is all about keeping your carbs low and increasing your fat intake?

For a lot of people just keeping low on carbs, helps in weight loss. However some people are more metabolically resistant than others and despite keeping their carb levels below 20 grams per day continue to gain weight. It is in such cases worth looking at your protein intake.

We give little attention to how much protein we need to consume in order to stay in ketosis. Our body cannot make protein on its own and as such protein is an important macronutrient without which your body wouldn't be able to carry out the necessary tissue building and repair functions.

What is Gluconeogenesis?

It is worth understanding the process of gluconeogenesis here. It is a metabolic process by which our body produces glucose from noncarbohydrate sources – amino acids in protein being one of them.

Gluconeogenesis is an essential process without which we probably cannot survive for long, especially if we need to go without food. This is because our body needs a constant and steady flow of glucose to keep the brain and red blood cells functioning.

However when we consume more protein than our body needs the excess is turned into glucose. This glucose is over and above the minimum requirement of the body and results in weight gain.

Optimum Protein Intake

There are various theories on how you can calculate the ideal protein intake taking your weight in pounds and then multiple it by 0.6 and 1.0. This will then give you the ideal range for your protein intake in grams.

An easier way is to pick a level of protein and while still keeping carbs below 20 grams monitor how you are doing for that quantity of protein intake. If you continue to struggle, keep shifting your intake downwards till you hit the sweet spot.

It is worth noting that when you are experimenting to find your ideal level of protein intake you must keep your carbs low and have adequate monounsaturated and saturated fats to give you the much needed satiety.

If you are struggling with weight loss due to being more sensitive to proteins, try and avoid leaner cuts of meat like chicken breast as that would elevate your blood sugar levels and make you gain weight just by having too much protein than your body needs. On the other side, cuts of meats with saturated fat will automatically lower your protein intake and help in weight loss.

Mistake 11:

LIFESTYLE CHALLENGES

The biggest lifestyle failures that encourage binging and hence weight gain are stress and sleep deprivation. Let us examine both and understand how we can overcome them.

Stress leads to overeating

It is not enough to just eat right and exercise, chronic stress levels can prevent you from losing weight or even add up pounds. Every time you are stressed, your body releases adrenaline, the fight or flight hormone, which is meant to help with dangerous or unexpected situations like running away from a lion's attack.

In today's time we get an adrenaline rush when we have a bad day at work or when we have a fight. With the release of adrenaline in the blood stream there is an increase in the flow of oxygen and glucose to the brain and suppression of non-emergency functions like digestion.

This is our body's way to prepare for active fight or flight although in modern times this has a negative effect on our bodies as the focus shifts from important functions like immunity and digestion and overworks our heart with the increased oxygen supply.

We tend to feel hungry as our body, thinking it is in active survival mode, is made to believe that all the calories have been consumed in dealing with the stress when in reality we haven't. As a result we overeat.

At the same time our body releases stress hormone cortisol, which at chronically high levels will cause you to be hungry all the time and crave for unhealthy starchy carbs. These carbs particularly when combined with salt and fat (like in pizza, chips, cookies) trigger a reaction in our brain that provides a temporary relief to our feeling of being sad, low or anxious.

Meditation and deep breathing exercises help to reduce incidences of stress eating.

Sleep Deprivation

Once in awhile most of us stay up late at night to meet a project deadline or to catch up on a favourite soap opera. We all know that not getting enough sleep leaves us tired, irritable and less productive the next day.

However when you skimp on sleep on a regular basis, that's when the real problem starts. Being chronically sleep deprived produces less growth hormone, slows down glucose metabolism and decreases the level of leptin – the satiety hormone.

So you feel hungry, are not satisfied after a meal and crave for carbs all the time. Lack of sleep also increases the production of ghrelin in the gut – the hormone that signals the brain when we are hungry.

When you are not getting enough sleep the chances are high that your brain will try to make up for the low energy by increasing the intake of food and you will eat more than you need to. Also, as you are low on leptin you will not know when to stop eating. So you eat when you don't need to and eat lot more than your body requires.

You should attempt to get at least seven hours of sleep at night and minimize screen time just before going to bed. This will help you in unwinding at night. Also, keeping your alcohol levels in check at night will help improve the quality of sleep.

Mistake 12:

FALLING FOR FAKE PRODUCTS

Wouldn't it be great if we could eat bread, pasta and chocolate and still lose weight rapidly without hunger or all the complicated diseases associated with sugar?

There are plenty of shady businesses that promise the impossible. An excellent example is low carb pasta from Dreamfields, which tastes like any regular pasta. They are even made from regular starchy wheat, but the manufacturer still claims that our body does not absorb the carbs as their pasta is protected from some *"patent pending process"*.

The problem is that their claims are completely bogus and raises blood sugar like any regular pasta. Based on several researches it was proved that their pasta behaved like regular pasta and Dreamfields had to pay a settlement fine of $ 8 million because they had lied.

However by then they had sold their fake low carb pasta for 10 years.

There are many similar examples of fake products. Carbzone is a company that claims to be selling low carb products. They claim their tortilla made from whole wheat is low carb, however on testing it showed to contain 3 times as many carbs as stated on the label.

Even low carb chocolate cookies from the Atkins Company often contain sugar alcohol like maltitol, which the maker pretends to not raise blood sugar. However this claim has no merit and about half of it does end up raising blood sugar. The manufactures omit sugar alcohols from the net carb count, so that they can market it as low carb.

In short, do not fall for fake products. If it tastes like bread, pasta or chocolate then the reality is that it is bread, pasta and chocolate.

Frequently Asked Questions

Still have some unanswered questions about the ketogenic diet? Below we have tried to address some of the commonly asked questions on the diet.

Pre-diet

For those embarking on the Ketogenic Diet for the first time, you may have a lot of questions before you start. Luckily, we have the answers to your most frequently asked questions below!

Is Ketogenic Diet Right for Me?

Ketogenic Diet is great for people who want to lose weight and improve their overall health. It's also a good choice for diabetics as a way of controlling their insulin levels.

Can Vegetarians do Keto?

Yes! Vegetarian can enjoy ketogenic diet, but will obviously have to supplement or replace some foods. Eggs and dairy can be great substitutes for meat, as can green vegetables such as broccoli.

Can I Still Drink Coffee?

Yes. Coffee is low in carbohydrates so you can drink it while following ketogenic diet.

What if My Doctor says Low-Carb is Junk Science?

Many doctors are not nutritionists and so they lack the proper training to advise on ketogenic diet. Unfortunately there is an old fashioned perception which many physicians still believe, that low fat equals weight loss rather than low carb. At the end of the day, many followers of Ketogenic Diet have seen weight loss and improved health.

Is Cheating Worth It?

Ketogenic Diet has been proven to promote weight loss and improve health, but, like any healthy eating program, it only works if you stick to it and follow the core principles of the diet.

Keto Adaptation

It stands to reason that when you change your diet you will encounter some adaption issues, so here we round up and explain some of the most common worries.

Adaptation Period & Keto Flu

When starting ketogenic diet, most people will go through what is known as "keto flu". Actually this is nothing to do with the flu virus and is just your body's natural reaction to cutting out carbohydrates.

Please don't panic and think that Ketogenic Diet is not good for you if this happens. The symptoms of "keto flu" like tiredness, nausea and dizziness. Keto flu can be combated by upping your electrolyte intake and it should pass within a few days.

Help, I'm in Keto and I Never Poop! What do I do?

Some people who start Ketogenic Diet forget that you need to eat a balanced diet from different food groups and not just meat and dairy, which can lead to constipation. If you find this is an issue try to up your vegetable and nut intake and drink plenty of water. Include more good fats like avocado and coconut oil in your daily meals.

Eating Too Many Nuts and Dairy

There is a great misunderstanding about whether you should eat nuts and dairy on Ketogenic Diet and the answer is yes as long as it is in moderation. When most followers start a ketogenic diet, they end up eating too much dairy and nuts, which are high in calories but low in carbs. Overeating these would lead to your weight loss goals stalling. The best tip is to eat nuts and dairy as part of a mix of food groups.

Lifestyle challenges

Now that we have looked at the adaptation issues for those embarking on ketogenic diet, let's look at the lifestyle challenges that some followers may face. We will also look at the best ways that these can be addressed.

Keto on a Budget

Some people worry about following Ketogenic Diet on a budget. But actually once you start, you'll find that your monthly spend on food will actually go down. This is because

- You will buy fresh base ingredients instead of processed ingredients
- Once you hit ketosis, you will observe that satiety comes much earlier and you will eat less. This is another sign that you are in the state of Ketosis.

Farmers market is a great place to shop for fresh ingredients while on Keto. You will find pocket friendly bargains there while supporting the local community. Moreover you will learn more about your food by being in direct touch with the producers. I have personally learnt so much by interacting with the farmers in these weekly markets.

Eating Out

Eating in a restaurant can seem daunting when you first start following ketogenic diet. Actually it doesn't need to be difficult if you follow a few simple rules.

Firstly, try to stick to meat, dairy, or vegetable dishes that don't come with rice, pasta, or bread. Things like steak with salad are a good choice, as are salads on their own with cheese or meat added. Other good choices when eating out can be fish or seafood with non-starchy vegetables.

Just be careful to have them with olive oil rather than dressings, which can be high in sugar. Also remember that it is up to you if you want to customize your order and ask for things like sauces to be left out, so don't be afraid to ask!

It also is worth checking with the restaurants if they have Keto/Paleo/LCHF friendly dishes.

Eating with Friends and Family

Friends and family may not understand Ketogenic Diet and may want you to eat whatever they are eating, especially if you have done so in the past. At the end of the day, you may not be able to explain the principles of Ketogenic Diet to them in a way that changes their minds, but just remember that it is up to you to choose what to eat. They may just be convinced when they see your weight loss and renewed energy levels!

Weight Maintenance

One of the big questions when it comes to starting and maintaining Ketogenic Diet is how to control weight loss and establish a healthy goal weight and then stick to it! These are all great questions and here we break down normal weight loss patterns for followers of Keto Diet and how to address them.

Help! Why have I plateaued?

Keto Diet is an effective way of losing weight, but if not followed correctly it can lead to weight plateau. There are a few reasons why this can happen on Keto Diet.

Water Weight

Weight loss plateau can happen in about week 2 or 3 of people starting on the diet.Everyone reacts differently, and many people lose a lot of weight initially, much of which is water weight. This is perfectly normal and healthy and once the water weight comes off, it can take time for your body to start losing fat.

Followers of Ketogenic Diet need to understand this process and make sure they give their new diet time to take effect.

Still Burning Glucose

You could still be burning glucose if you still have a high carbohydrate intake, either because of 'cheating days' when you eat carbs or because you don't properly identify which foods have a high carb count.

Secondly for weight plateau may be because you are eating too much protein, which inhibits ketosis as we discussed earlier.

The best way to combat this is keep an eye on your food intake to make sure that you are eating the right balance of macronutrients.

I've Reached my Goal Weight, Now What?

Congratulations! Once you reach your goal weight then one of the best things you can do is use a keto calculator [9] which will calculate the ideal levels of carbs and protein you can now eat in order to stay at your desired weight.

What do I Need to Know about Intermittent Fasting and Fat Fasting?

Intermittent fasting is when you choose certain periods such as a time of day or a full day itself to fast and refrain from any food intake. Weight loss studies that go as far back as the 1950s have shown that fasting helps weight loss and boosts your body's ability to burn fat [10]

The only difference between intermittent fasting and fat fasting is that the first one cuts out all food groups and the second works on the premise that you will eat 80-90% of your total daily calories from fat while at the same time only ingesting 1,000-1,200 calories a day.

Both of these fasts are known to speed up weight loss, especially if one is experiencing a weight plateau, although it should not be used until you have been on Keto Diet for at least 4 weeks and have achieved ketosis.

I'm on Keto Diet but I'm bored!

Some followers of Keto Diet feel like they are just eating the same kinds of foods every day, which can lead to boredom and make it easy to fall off the Keto Diet wagon.

If this happens to you remember that there are a wide range of food recipes available online. One great way to get some inspiration is to recipe swap with other followers of Keto Diet so that you expand your culinary repertoire.

Another fantastic way to ensure that you switch things up is to follow the seasons and focus on buying seasonal produce. This means that you will not only be cooking the freshest and best ingredients available but you also won't get a chance to be bored before another exciting new ingredient comes into season bringing with it a whole range of new recipe ideas!

Also do your best to plan meals ahead, as last minute cooking can lead to the same quick and easy recipes which may be healthy but can get a little dull when you eat them every day.

Focus on cooking a different dish for each day of the week as well as switching up your snack choices and dessert options. This should help you stay interested and motivated.

Conclusion

Thanks again for downloading this book!

I hope this book was able to help you lose weight and live a healthier life. If you want my personal **Keto Meal Plan** and my **Everyday Keto Tips** please write to me at kindlehealthnbeauty@gmail.com

Finally, if you enjoyed this book, then I'd like to ask you for a favour, would you be kind enough to leave a review for this book on Amazon? It'd be greatly appreciated!

Please leave a review for this book on Amazon!

Thank you and Happy Keto Dieting!

Resources

External Links

1. http://www.nejm.org/doi/full/10.1056/NEJMoa022637
2. http://nutritionandmetabolism.biomedcentral.com/articles/10.1186/1743-7075-2-31
3. http://www.ncbi.nlm.nih.gov/pubmed/19082851
4. http://ajcn.nutrition.org/content/87/1/44.full
5. http://nutritionandmetabolism.biomedcentral.com/articles/10.1186/1743-7075-1-13
6. http://www.ncbi.nlm.nih.gov/pmc/articles/PMC2367001
7. http://link.springer.com/article/10.1007%2Fs10620-006-9433-5
8. www.ketodietapp.com
9. Keto calculator
10. Kekwick, A., and Pawan, L.S., "Calorie Intake in Relation to Body Weight Changes in the Obese", Lancet, 1956.

Books

- Fat Chance
- Why we get Fat
- The Obesity Code

Top Keto Blogs

http://www.ruled.me/
https://mindliftingmouthgasms.com/
http://www.ketogenic-diet-resource.com/
http://mariamindbodyhealth.com/
http://www.marksdailyapple.com/
http://thenourishedcaveman.com/
http://www.tasteaholics.com/
http://alldayidreamaboutfood.com/

List of 56 names of Sugar

Sugar / Sucrose
High Fructose corn syrup
Agave Nectar
Beet sugar
Blackstrap molasses
Brown sugar
Buttered syrup
Cane juice crystals
Cane sugar
Caramel
Carob syrup
Castor sugar
Coconut Sugar
Confectioner's sugar
(powdered sugar)
Date sugar
Demerara sugar
Evaporated cane juice
Florida crystals
Fruit Juice
Fruit juice concentrate
Golden sugar
Golden syrup
Grape sugar
Honey
Icing sugar
Invert sugar
Maple Syrup
Molasses

Muscovado sugar
Panela sugar
Raw sugar
Refiner's syrup
Sorghum syrup
Sucanat
Treacle sugar
Turbinado sugar
Yellow sugar
Barley malt
Brown rice syrup
Corn syrup
Corn syrup solids
Dextrin
Dextrose
Diastatic malt
Ethyl maltol
Glucose
Glucose solids
Lactose
Malt syrup
Maltodextrin
Maltose
Rice syrup
Crystalline fructose
Fructose
D-ribose
Galactose

Foods to Eat and Avoid

When you are following Ketogenic Diet you need to avoid all foods that are high in carbohydrates or contain sugar. This means cutting out:

- Foods with high starch content: Products that contain wheat including pasta, rice, and cereal. This also includes other grains.
- Beans and legumes including all beans, peas, lentils, and chickpeas.
- Fruit with the exception of some berries in small quantities like blueberries.
- Foods containing Sugar: Ice cream, candy, cakes, cookies, soda, and even fruit juice and smoothies.
- Condiments and sauces like salad dressings or barbecue sauce.
- Products that are Low Fat and processed as these are high in carbs.
- All root vegetables like potatoes, sweet potatoes, carrots, and parsnips.
- Unhealthy fats like vegetable oils, trans fats and oils rich in omega 6.
- Sugar Free or Diet Foods as these are highly processed.

On the flipside, foods that you should eat as part of Ketogenic Diet include:

- All types of meat including beef, chicken, turkey, and pork.
- Oily and fatty fish such as tuna, salmon, mackerel, and trout.
- Eggs- They contain plenty of omega-3.
- Butter and cream, particularly from animals that have been grass fed.
- Nuts and seeds.
- Unprocessed cheese like goat, cheddar, or mozzarella.
- Healthy fats like coconut oil, avocado oil, or extra virgin olive oil.
- Avocados.
- Green vegetables or vegetables that are low in carbs like tomatoes, onions, and peppers.
- Condiments like salt, pepper, or spices.

45005948R00032

Made in the USA
San Bernardino, CA
29 January 2017